The Plant Power Diet

The Plant Power Diet

TRANSFORM YOUR HEALTH WITH
NATURE'S BOUNTY,

B. Vincent

QuantumQuill Press

Contents

Introduction   1

1 Chapter 1: The Basics of Plant-Based Nutrition   4

2 Chapter 2: Getting Started with the Plant Power Diet   8

3 Chapter 3: Optimizing Nutrition on a Plant-Based Diet   13

4 Chapter 4: Overcoming Challenges and Staying Motivated   18

5 Chapter 5: Beyond Nutrition: The Environmental and Ethical Impacts   24

6 Chapter 6: Advanced Plant-Based Nutrition   30

7 Chapter 7: The Future of Food: Trends and Innovations   37

Conclusion: Embracing the Plant Power Lifestyle   43

First Printing, 2024

Introduction

Prologue to Plant-Based Sustenance

Welcome to the extraordinary universe of plant-based sustenance — a domain where your food supports your body as well as safeguards the planet and regards all types of life. At its center, a plant-based diet is established in the utilization of vegetables, natural products, entire grains, vegetables, nuts, and seeds. These food sources structure the underpinning of feasts that are wealthy in supplements, fiber, and phytochemicals, the normal mixtures that plants produce to safeguard themselves and end up having critical medical advantages for us.

The advantages of embracing a plant-based way of life reach out a long ways past the individual. Logical exploration reliably demonstrates the way that such an eating regimen can bring down the gamble of creating coronary illness, hypertension, diabetes, and particular sorts of disease. It can likewise help with weight the executives and work on in general essentialness. Be that as it may, the effect of picking plant-based food varieties comes to further, adding to ecological manageability by lessening our carbon impression and saving water. An approach to eating lines up with a developing consciousness of what our decisions mean for our general surroundings.

Besides, taking on a plant-based diet is a stage towards a more merciful way of life. It shakes things up of creature farming, featuring a way towards lessening animal torment. By picking plants over creature items, we offer a quiet expression against rehearses that we probably shouldn't uphold.

In setting out on this excursion, you could contemplate whether such an eating routine can give every one of the fundamental supplements your body needs. Allow me to console you: with smart preparation, a plant-based diet can meet all your healthful necessities. This book is intended to direct you through understanding these wholesome establishments, guaranteeing that you can partake in a fluctuated, heavenly, and restorative eating regimen that upholds your prosperity as well as the strength of our planet and its occupants.

As we dive further into this book, remember that changing to a plant-based diet is an excursion. There's really no need with focus on flawlessness or complying to severe guidelines. About settling on decisions adjust all the more intimately with your qualities and your wellbeing objectives. Whether you're making your most memorable strides towards a plant-based diet or looking to extend your responsibility, this book is here to help you constantly. Welcome to the start of a groundbreaking excursion with the force of plants.

Manual for Utilizing This Book

Leaving on the excursion of plant-based sustenance is an interesting and extraordinary undertaking. This book is your compass, intended to explore you through the change easily and certainty. Whether you're totally new to plant-based eating or hoping to extend your comprehension and responsibility, we've organized this manual for meet you where you are and take you where you wish to go.

Bit by bit: We start with the rudiments — what a plant-based diet involves, its advantages, and how to guarantee it meets generally your wholesome necessities. Every part expands upon the last, directing you through the reasonable parts of taking on a plant-based way of life. From setting up your kitchen and understanding nourishment to dominating dinner arranging and planning, we cover everything.

Pragmatic Tips and Apparatuses: Past hypothesis, this book is loaded with down to earth counsel. You'll track down shopping records, dinner prep procedures, and ways to eat out. We figure out the difficulties that accompany changing your eating routine, so we offer answers for normal snags and how to conquer them.

Recipes and Motivation: What's information without application? Sprinkled all through the book are not difficult to-follow, tasty recipes that take special care of different preferences and inclinations. These recipes are something beyond fuel; they're intended to move euphoria and imagination in your plant-based venture.

Local area and Backing: Recall, progressing to a plant-based diet isn't just about changing what's on your plate; it's tied in with turning out to be essential for a more extensive local area of similar people. In the last sections, we investigate ways of associating with others on this way, sharing assets and stages where you can track down help, motivation, and fellowship.

This book isn't about inflexible principles or authoritative opinion. It's about investigation, learning, and development. As you turn these pages, we welcome you to keep a receptive outlook and heart. Take what impacts you, and feel free to as you go. Your plant-based venture is interestingly yours, and how you explore it ought to line up with your own objectives, wellbeing requirements, and way of life.

We're here to help you in finding the force of plant-based sustenance. We should leave on this excursion together, towards a better you and a more maintainable world. Welcome to "The Plant Power Diet: Change Your Wellbeing with Nature's Abundance."

1

Chapter 1: The Basics of Plant-Based Nutrition

Sustaining Preparations of Plant-Based Eating

Leaving on a plant-based adventure invites us to rethink what we eat, yet the manner by which we feed our bodies. At the center of plant-based sustenance is a clear, yet critical rule: nature offers a flood of food assortments copious in the supplements, minerals, and enhancements principal for enthusiastic prosperity. In this part, we dive into the feeding foundations that help a thriving plant-based lifestyle.

Plants are rockin' rollers of food. They are our fundamental well-springs of supplements, minerals, disease avoidance specialists, fiber, and phytonutrients — escalates that work synergistically to propel prosperity and defend against ailment. An especially organized plant-based diet can meet all your fortifying necessities, offering a balance of macronutrients (starches, proteins, and fats) close by an alternate group of micronutrients.

Protein, much of the time a mark of combination of feeding discussions, is bounteous in the plant domain. Vegetables, nuts, seeds, whole grains, and even vegetables add to a complete amino destructive profile when consumed over the course of a day. Understanding how to join these sources ensures that your protein needs are met, supporting all that from muscle fix and improvement to impetus and substance creation.

Fats are major for frontal cortex prosperity, supplement osmosis, and cell ability. Picking plant-based wellsprings of fat, similar to avocados, nuts, seeds, and olives, gives your body heart-strong monounsaturated and polyunsaturated fats, including omega-3 unsaturated fats fundamental for mental and cardiovascular prosperity.

Sugars, the body's fundamental energy source, should come from whole, normal plant food assortments like natural items, vegetables, and whole grains. These food assortments give the fiber essential to stomach related prosperity, help with overseeing glucose levels, and add to a vibe of finish and satisfaction after feasts.

Micronutrients, including supplements and minerals, are plentiful in a varied plant-based diet. Faint blended greens, for example, are copious in calcium, iron, and vitamin K, while food varieties developed from the beginning all tones give a scope of supplements, minerals, and cell fortifications. Understanding which food sources are rich in unambiguous enhancements licenses you to accommodate your eating routine to meet your own prosperity needs.

A common concern is the openness of explicit enhancements, similar to Vitamin B12, Vitamin D, and Omega-3 unsaturated fats, which are regularly associated with animal things. Fortunately, fortified food sources and improvements can ensure adequate confirmation of these enhancements, making it possible to stay aware of ideal prosperity on a plant-based diet.

In overview, a plant-based diet, when well organized, isn't simply restoratively adequate yet can in like manner be particularly prosperity progressing. It invites us to research the assortment of plant food sources, each with its striking supporting profile, to make an eating schedule that maintains life, criticalness, and success. As we adventure through this segment, we'll sort out some way to harness the dietary power of plants to fuel our bodies and backing our spirits.

Clinical benefits of Plant-Based Diets

The shift towards a plant-based diet conveys with it a cornucopia of clinical benefits, endorsed by a consistently creating gathering of legitimate assessment. This segment dives into how taking on an eating routine in view of regular items, vegetables, whole grains, vegetables, nuts, and seeds can be an exceptional power for our prosperity, offering protection against different ailments and working on our physical and mental flourishing.

Heart Prosperity: The heart is the underpinning of our prosperity, and a plant-based diet is perhaps of its best accomplice. Studies have dependably shown that the people who take on plant-driven consumes less calories have a lower risk of making coronary sickness. The reasons are mind boggling; such weight control plans are ordinarily lower in submerged fats and cholesterol, while being well off in fiber and heart-sound enhancements like potassium, magnesium, and cell fortifications. These parts participate to lessen circulatory strain, further foster cholesterol levels, and work on the overall sufficiency of our veins.

Diabetes Contravention and The chiefs: The overall rising in diabetes has been met with certain verification that a plant-based diet can offer tremendous benefits in hindering and managing the disorder. By propelling a strong weight, further creating insulin responsiveness, and offering a low glycemic load, plant-based diets can help with offsetting glucose levels and may reduce the prerequisite for solution in individuals with type 2 diabetes.

Weight The chiefs: Strength is a crushing prosperity concern, but one that a plant-based diet can help address. Food assortments that are staples in a plant-based diet are generally lower in calories anyway higher in fiber and volume, adding to impressions of finishing and satisfaction without the excess calories. This can regularly incite weight decrease and upkeep without the prerequisite for calorie counting or restrictive dietary examples.

Steady Disease Balance: Past coronary sickness and diabetes, a plant-based diet offers protection against a scope of diligent conditions. From decreasing the bet of explicit threatening developments to shielding against mental debasement, the enhancements found in plant food sources can expect a fundamental part in thwarting disease. The quieting and disease counteraction specialist properties of plant-based food sources are key supporters, offering our bodies protection at the telephone level.

In this segment, we'll examine these benefits all the more carefully, emptying the frameworks by which a plant-based diet maintains our prosperity and how doing the switch can provoke huge changes in our flourishing. Through understanding the significant clinical benefits of plant-based sustenance, we can see the worth in the power of our dietary choices for of food, yet as a gadget for disorder countering and prosperity improvement.

2

～

Chapter 2: Getting Started with the Plant Power Diet

Laying out Your Objectives

Leaving on a plant-based venture is similar as setting out on any incredible experience — it starts with characterizing where you need to go. The initial step isn't in the kitchen, nor is it in the supermarket passageways; it's inside yourself, understanding your inspirations and what you plan to accomplish. This section guides you through setting smart, individual wellbeing objectives that are dreams as well as objections you can reach.

Find Your Why: Each excursion has a beginning stage, and in the domain of plant-based eating, it starts with a straightforward inquiry: Why? Maybe you're propelled by a longing for better wellbeing, ecological worries, or moral reasons connected with creature government assistance. Recognizing your center inspiration is essential; it will be the compass that keeps you situated toward your objectives, particularly when difficulties emerge.

Laying out Brilliant Objectives: The idea of Shrewd objectives — Explicit, Quantifiable, Feasible, Important, and Time-bound — gives a system to setting goals that are clear and reachable inside a predefined time period. For example, as opposed to a dubious desire like "eat better," a Brilliant objective would be "integrate no less than three distinct sorts of vegetables into my dinners every day for the following month." This approach guarantees your objectives are unmistakable and identifiable.

Making an Arrangement: With your objectives set, the following stage is making an arrangement to accomplish them. This could include instructing yourself about plant-based sustenance, arranging your dinners, or tracking down a local area of similar people for help. Your arrangement ought to frame noteworthy advances that continuously draw you nearer to your objective, considering adaptability and advancing en route.

Expecting Difficulties: Changing to a plant-based diet isn't without its obstacles. Whether it's exploring social circumstances or tending to dietary worries, expecting these difficulties permits you to plan arrangements ahead of time. For instance, figuring out how to find plant-based choices while feasting out or understanding how to adjust your supplement admission can assist with smoothing your way.

In defining your objectives for embracing a plant-based diet, recall that this excursion is yours alone. Your speed, your inspirations, and the particular goals you set are private to you. This part is intended to furnish you with the instruments and certainty expected to lay out significant objectives and make a guide for accomplishing them. By finding opportunity to reflect and design, you're establishing the groundwork for an effective and feasible progress to plant-based living.

Kitchen Makeover

Changing your eating routine starts with changing the very space where your food processes start: your kitchen. A kitchen makeover is something other than a cleaning binge; it's tied in with adjusting your current circumstance to your new plant-based objectives. This part will direct you through making a kitchen that backings as well as motivates your plant-based way of life.

Cleansing Non-Plant-Based Things: The most important phase in your kitchen makeover is to get out things that never again line up with your plant-based objectives. This doesn't be guaranteed to mean waste; consider giving unopened things to nearby food banks or imparting to loved ones. The point is to account for new, empowering fixings that will frame the premise of your plant-based dinners.

Loading Up on Fundamentals: A plant-fueled kitchen is supplied with different entire, natural food varieties. Entire grains like quinoa, earthy colored rice, and oats; vegetables like lentils, chickpeas, and dark beans; a variety of flavors and spices; nuts and seeds; and, obviously, a lot of new foods grown from the ground. These staples offer dietary lavishness as well as adaptability in cooking.

Putting resources into Key Kitchen Apparatuses: Certain instruments can make plant-based cooking more effective and agreeable. A top notch blender is fundamental for smoothies, soups, and sauces. A food processor deals with cleaving and dicing, as well as making nut margarines and falafel. Other supportive instruments incorporate a decent arrangement of blades, different cutting sheets, and capacity compartments for dinner prep and extras.

Arranging for Straightforwardness and Availability: What you coordinate your kitchen can incredibly mean for your dinner arrangement proficiency. Place the food varieties and hardware you utilize most frequently in simple to-arrive at places. Sorting out your storage space and cooler by food classifications not just assists with regards to following of what you have yet additionally in igniting dinner thoughts. A methodical kitchen welcomes innovativeness and diminishes the pressure of dinner prep.

By giving your kitchen a plant-based makeover, you're making way for progress. This change isn't just about eliminating what you can't have however, more significantly, about praising and making available the wealth of food sources that you can appreciate. With a kitchen that reflects your wellbeing desires, you're prepared to set out on this excursion of revelation and sustenance.

Straightforward and Nutritious Recipes

The core of the plant-based venture lies in the dinners you make — dishes that are nutritious as well as welcoming and scrumptious. This segment is your gold mine of straightforward, nutritious recipes that make the plant-based diet available and agreeable, in any event, for those simply beginning. Whether you're cooking for one, for a family, or for companions distrustful of plant-based eating, these recipes are intended to please and fulfill.

Breakfast Enjoyments: Start your day with invigorating dinners that set an inspirational vibe. Investigate recipes for smoothies loaded with natural products, vegetables, and plant-based proteins that prepare you for the day ahead. Find the straightforwardness of short-term oats, adaptable with your number one garnishes, or flavorful choices like tofu scramble that demonstrate breakfast can be both generous and plant-based.

Snacks to Anticipate: Lunch is an amazing chance to refuel with lively, supplement thick feasts. Dig into recipes for generous plates of mixed greens that go past lettuce and carrot, consolidating grains, beans, and a rainbow of vegetables. Figure out how to get ready wraps and sandwiches loaded up with delightful spreads and a wealth of new, crunchy vegetables. These feasts are ideally suited for in a hurry eating or a fantastic late morning break.

Suppers that Joy: Night dinners are a chance to loosen up and partake in the delights of cooking and eating. This segment incorporates recipes for ameliorating soups, stews, and curries that stew with the kinds of plants. Find how to make plant-based adaptations of natural top picks, like lasagna or tacos, utilizing imaginative, empowering fixings. Every recipe is made in all honestly, guaranteeing you invest less energy in the kitchen and additional time appreciating your manifestations.

Bites and Sides: Finishing our culinary excursion are the additional items that make eating a delight — 'tidbits and side dishes. From fresh prepared kale chips to smooth, velvety hummus, these recipes give solid choices to nibbling or supplementing any dinner. Get familiar with the craft of making side dishes that can raise a straightforward feast to something uniquely great, as simmered root vegetables or a quinoa salad overflowing with flavors.

Every recipe inside this assortment is in excess of a bunch of guidelines; it's a challenge to examination and track down delight during the time spent cooking. By zeroing in on straightforwardness and nourishment, these recipes demystify plant-based cooking, making it open to everybody, no matter what their culinary ability level. As you investigate and taste, you'll find that plant-based eating isn't about limitation yet about praising the overflow and assortment that nature offers.

3

Chapter 3: Optimizing Nutrition on a Plant-Based Diet

Protein Power

One of the most broadly perceived questions looked by those leaving on a plant-based diet is, "Where do you get your protein?" This part is focused on scattering the legend that plant-based consumes less calories can't give adequate protein to ideal prosperity. Protein is fundamental for the body's abilities, including muscle fix, advancement, and the upkeep of strong skin, hair, and nails. Fortunately, the plant domain is plentiful in protein-rich food assortments, offering different sources to meet and outperform your everyday necessities.

Understanding Plant-Based Proteins: Not in any way shape or form like animal sources, plant proteins offer a total heap of fiber, supplements, minerals, and cell fortifications, with the extra benefit of being low in submerged fats. Vegetables — like lentils, chickpeas, and dull beans — are powerhouses of protein, fiber, and iron. Nuts and seeds, including almonds, chia seeds, and hemp seeds, give protein as well as sound fats and omega-3 unsaturated fats. Whole grains like quinoa, grain, and bulgur wheat also contribute gigantic protein to the eating schedule, close by major B supplements and fiber.

Coordinating Plant Proteins into Banquets: This segment offers helpful guidance on the most capable strategy to consolidate a combination of plant-based proteins in your everyday meals. Breakfast can be invigorated with a smoothie upgraded with pea protein powder or a bowl of oats polished off with nuts and seeds. Lunch and dinner can incorporate great plates of leafy greens, soups, and stews spun around beans and lentils, or whole grains filling in as a base for various enhancements and sauces.

Solidifying Proteins for Complete Sustenance: While it was once acknowledged that plant-based eaters expected to carefully join proteins at each banquet to shape a 'complete' protein, we at present understand that the body can pool the amino acids it needs all through the range of the day. In any case, this part really includes the upsides of merging different plant proteins to ensure an alternate confirmation of amino acids, which can overhaul by and large balance and savor the experience of meals.

Tending to Protein Needs: Whether you're a contender with higher protein needs or someone expecting to stay aware of general prosperity, this part provides guidance on determining your protein essentials and meeting them through plant-based sources. With an assortment of protein-rich plants accessible to you, achieving your protein goals isn't simply possible anyway can in like manner be a tasty and satisfying aspect of your eating routine.

Close to the completion of this part, you'll have a broad perception of the plentiful protein sources open in a plant-based diet and how to coordinate them into your banquets creatively and effectively. With this data, the protein question will at this point not be a concern yet an opportunity to examine the sumptuousness of plant-based food.

Fats: The Incomparable and the Indispensable

In the trip of understanding plant-based food, the subject of fats stands firm on a footing of essential importance. This part hopes to illuminate the occupation of strong fats in a fair plant-based diet, scattering dreams that all fats are foes. In reality, fats are key for different actual cycles, including mind prosperity, compound creation, and the maintenance of fat-dissolvable supplements. Plus, they add a magnificent abundance to suppers, updating both flavor and satiety.

The Meaning of Sound Fats: Isolating between such fats is dire. While drenched and trans fats, oftentimes found in animal things and dealt with food assortments, can add to coronary sickness and other clinical issues, unsaturated fats expect an important part in our eating schedule. These heart-sound fats, including monounsaturated and polyunsaturated fats, support by and large when consumed with some restriction.

Wellsprings of Plant-Based Fats: This part directs you through the best wellsprings of plant-based fats. Avocados, for example, are affluent in monounsaturated fats as well as stacked with fiber and potassium. Nuts and seeds, similar to walnuts, flaxseeds, and chia seeds, give omega-3 unsaturated fats, basic for mind ability and diminishing bothering. Nut margarines offer a supportive and tasty strategy for coordinating these fats into your eating routine. Also, oils like olive oil and avocado oil can be used in cooking to add sound fats and flavor to dishes.

Changing Omega-3 and Omega-6 Unsaturated fats: Achieving the right concordance between omega-3 and omega-6 unsaturated fats is crucial for hindering bothering and progressing overall prosperity. This part offers methods for changing these principal fats, underlining the meaning of extending omega-3 confirmation through flaxseeds, chia seeds, hemp seeds, and green development based upgrades to adjust the routinely higher omega-6 substance in the state of the art diet.

Coordinating Strong Fats into Your Eating routine: Practical direction on the most capable strategy to integrate sound fats into your regular meals ensures that you can participate in the upsides of these basic enhancements. From adding avocado to your morning smoothie to sprinkling seeds on your plates of leafy greens and coordinating nuts into nibbles and treats, there are huge approaches to further developing your eating routine with plant-based fats.

As we wrap up this part, you'll have gained an extensive cognizance of the essential work fats play in a plant-based diet. You'll be outfitted with the data to seek after informed choices about coordinating strong fats into your blowouts, it is anyway supporting as it is by all accounts wonderful to ensure your eating routine. With this foundation, you're very much made a beeline for further developing your plant-based sustenance for vigorous prosperity.

Supplements and Minerals

Setting out on a plant-based adventure conveys with it the commitment to promise one's eating routine is stacked with the significant supplements and minerals for ideal prosperity. This part is given to demystifying the principal micronutrients that are regularly highlighted as stresses for those taking on a plant-based lifestyle. Through understanding and key arrangement, you can ensure your plant-based diet is refreshingly wrapped up.

Key Enhancements of Focus: Among the enhancements habitually analyzed in plant-based swears off food are Vitamin B12, iron, calcium, and Vitamin D. These enhancements are essential for energy creation, oxygen transportation, bone prosperity, and resistant ability, independently. While it is really the situation that these enhancements are typically associated with animal things, this part will guide you through the plant-based sources and methods to ensure adequate confirmation.

Vitamin B12: Key for nerve ability and the improvement of DNA and red platelets, Vitamin B12 is the one enhancement not ordinarily available in plant food sources. This fragment looks at the meaning of strengthened food sources, for instance, certain plant milks, breakfast cereals, and empowering yeast, as well as the need of Vitamin B12 supplementation for those on a plant-based diet.

Iron: While plant-based diets can give above and beyond iron through food assortments like lentils, chickpeas, beans, tofu, and faint blended greens, the sort of iron in plants (non-heme iron) isn't exactly basically as quickly devoured as the heme iron found in animal things. This segment offers frameworks to overhaul iron maintenance, such as eating L-ascorbic corrosive rich food assortments nearby iron-rich food sources to increase iron take-up in a general sense.

Calcium and Vitamin D: Basic for bone prosperity, calcium, and vitamin D can be gotten from supported plant milks and crushes, faint serving of mixed greens, and specific kinds of tofu. The occupation of light in Vitamin D mixture is furthermore analyzed, nearby the proposition for Vitamin D improvements, especially in regions with less sun transparency.

Further developing Enhancement Ingestion: Past perceiving well-springs of these crucial enhancements, this segment gives tips to helping their maintenance. From feast sythesis to cooking techniques, little changes can overhaul the bioavailability of supplements and minerals, promising you get the best benefit from your plant-based meals.

Close to the completion of this segment, perusers will be furnished with the data and frameworks expected to unhesitatingly investigate the sustaining portions of a plant-based diet. Understanding how to meet your supplement and mineral necessities ensures the balance of needs as well as the upgrade of prosperity and flourishing on a plant-based adventure.

4

~

Chapter 4: Overcoming Challenges and Staying Motivated

Managing Social Circumstances

Exploring the social scene as a plant-based eater frequently presents one of the more nuanced challenges on this excursion. Whether it's a family assembling, a feast out with companions, or a working environment capability, these situations can here and there test your responsibility and require a smart methodology. This part is committed to furnishing you with procedures to effortlessly deal with these circumstances while remaining consistent with your plant-based values.

Planning is Critical: Prior to going to a get-together, pause for a minute to investigate the menu on the off chance that you're feasting out, or speak with your host assuming it's a confidential occasion. Numerous cafés are obliging of dietary inclinations, and a straightforward call ahead can guarantee there are plant-based choices accessible. For individual social occasions, proposing to bring a dish ensures you'll have something to eat as well as acquaints others with the enjoyments of plant-based cooking.

Imparting Your Necessities: With regards to examining your dietary decisions, lucidity and energy go far. Outlining your eating regimen regarding individual wellbeing, moral convictions, or natural worries can encourage understanding. Keep in mind, the objective isn't to change over however to convey; sharing your reasons in a non-fierce way welcomes exchange as opposed to discuss.

Taking care of Incredulity and Questions: Confronting suspicion or interest in your diet is normal. Arm yourself with information about plant-based sustenance to resolve normal inquiries and misinterpretations unhesitatingly. Your certainty and affirmation can divert these cooperations from challenges into open doors for sharing and instruction.

Embracing Adaptability: While remaining consistent with your standards, there might be times when adaptability can ease social collaborations. This doesn't mean undermining your qualities yet rather exploring circumstances with beauty. For example, in the event that a dish is made with a minor non-plant-based fixing, you could decide to zero in on the purpose behind the dinner as opposed to its outright immaculateness, particularly in settings where rejecting could cause huge uneasiness or offense.

This part digs further into every one of these techniques, giving genuine models and viable counsel to guarantee your plant-based venture is socially charming and satisfying. By planning for and exploring social circumstances with premonition and effortlessness, you can keep up with your dietary decisions without settling on your public activity, reinforcing your purpose and maybe in any event, moving others en route.

Overseeing Desires

The excursion towards a plant-based diet can some of the time feel like a difficult task against desires for non-plant-based food varieties. Whether it's a yearning for the recognizable taste of cheddar, the surface of meat, or just the comfort of inexpensive food, these desires are a characteristic piece of the progress. This section is intended to arm you with systems to comprehend, make due, and at last change these desires into open doors for more profound obligation to your plant-based way of life.

Figuring out Desires: Desires frequently come from various sources

— propensity, close to home associations, dietary lacks, or essentially the body's acclimation to new food sources. Perceiving the main driver of your hankering is the most vital phase in tending to it. This understanding can enable you to settle on decisions that line up with your objectives, as opposed to being driven by passing cravings.

Plant-Based Trades for Normal Desires: For each non-plant-based food you could long for, there's a plant-based elective that can fulfill that craving without undermining your responsibility. Hankering the richness of cheddar? Nourishing yeast, cashew cream, and avocado can offer that rich surface and flavor. Yearning for meat? Investigate the universe of lentils, beans, mushrooms, and plant-based meats intended to copy the taste and surface of creature items. This part gives an exhaustive manual for plant-based trades for normal desires, guaranteeing you have the devices to keep focused.

Changing Your Sense of taste: Progressing to a plant-based diet isn't just about supplanting non-plant-based food sources with plant-based ones; it's likewise about retraining your sense of taste to appreciate and pine for the kinds of plants. Step by step presenting different natural products, vegetables, grains, and vegetables into your dinners can grow your taste inclinations and diminish desires over the long haul. Methods for preparing and getting ready plant-based dishes in delightful and fulfilling ways are additionally covered, assisting with making plant-based food varieties your new standard.

Embracing Desires as Any open doors: Rather than survey desires as hindrances, this part urges you to consider them to be amazing open doors for imagination in the kitchen and for supporting your obligation to your wellbeing and values. Each longing for is an opportunity to investigate new food varieties, to study nourishment, and to reinforce your determination.

Toward the finish of this part, you'll have a tool compartment for overseeing desires such that upholds your plant-based venture. You'll comprehend that desires are not an indication of shortcoming but rather a characteristic piece of the interaction, and with the right methodologies, they can be explored effectively. Furnished with information, innovativeness, and a more profound comprehension of your own body's signs, you can forge ahead with your way with certainty, embracing each hankering as a stage towards a better, more supportable way of life.

Remaining Inspired

The way to a plant-based way of life is a remunerating venture, cleared with enhancements in wellbeing, commitments to natural manageability, and moral living. In any case, similar to any critical way of life change, it can introduce difficulties that test your inspiration. This section is devoted to giving you techniques to support your inspiration, guaranteeing that your plant-based venture is satisfying and persevering.

Setting Reasonable Assumptions: Understanding that flawlessness isn't the objective is vital in keeping a positive and sensible viewpoint. Slip-ups and misfortunes are essential for the educational experience. By setting attainable assumptions, you can celebrate progress as opposed to harp on defects, keeping inspiration high.

Observing Advancement: Perceive and praise your achievements, regardless of how little they might appear. Whether it's dominating another plant-based recipe, seeing upgrades in your wellbeing, or enduring a get-together with your dietary decisions unblemished, recognizing these accomplishments energizes your inspiration to proceed.

Returning to Your "Why": Your explanations behind picking a plant-based way of life are the bedrock of your inspiration. Consistently helping yourself to remember these reasons — be it for wellbeing, natural, or moral contemplations — can revive your responsibility, particularly during testing times. Keeping a diary, making a dream board, or imparting your excursion to others can act as strong tokens of your "why."

Tracking down Local area and Backing: Leaving on a plant-based excursion can feel disconnecting on occasion, especially in the event that your group of friends doesn't share your dietary decisions. Searching out a local area — whether on the web or face to face — of similar people can offer priceless help, motivation, and a feeling of having a place. Sharing encounters, difficulties, and triumphs with other people who comprehend your process can support your inspiration and give new points of view.

In this part, we dive into these methodologies exhaustively, offering commonsense tips and genuine guides to assist you with remaining propelled on your plant-based venture. From figuring out how to embrace the excursion's high points and low points to finding euphoria during the time spent disclosure and development, these procedures are intended to keep you propelled and focused on your plant-based way of life.

Keep in mind, the excursion to plant-based living is as much about the actual excursion for what it's worth about the objective. By remaining persuaded and embracing the excursion with an open heart and psyche, you'll find that the prizes stretch out a long ways past the food on your plate, enhancing your life in manners you might in all likelihood never have envisioned.

Examples of overcoming adversity

Setting out on a plant-based venture is a profoundly private undertaking, yet the difficulties confronted and triumphs accomplished frequently resound generally among the individuals who have picked this way. This section is a gathering of persuasive examples of overcoming adversity from people who have embraced a plant-based diet as well as have flourished as a result of it. Their stories act as strong demonstrations of the groundbreaking capability of plant-based living, giving inspiration, knowledge, and consolation to perusers at any phase of their excursion.

Various Excursions, Shared objectives: Every story starts with a foundation of the singular's life before their progress to a plant-based diet, featuring the different inspirations that motivated their change — be it wellbeing concerns, moral reasons, or natural contemplations. These accounts highlight the way that there is not a great explanation to set out on this way, and that everybody's process is special.

Challenges Survive: Fundamental to these accounts is the sincere sharing of difficulties looked en route. From exploring social circumstances and relational intricacies to beating desires and learning better approaches to cook and eat, these accounts dive into the real factors of making a huge way of life shift. All the more significantly, they share the techniques, mentalities, and emotionally supportive networks that assisted them with defeating these obstacles, offering pragmatic counsel and fortitude to perusers confronting comparative difficulties.

Changes Saw: The core of every story is the change experienced — upgrades in wellbeing measurements, (for example, weight, cholesterol levels, and pulse), improved physical and mental prosperity, and a more profound association with moral and natural qualities. These changes are not recently told; they are appeared through private stories, making the advantages of a plant-based diet distinctive and engaging.

Useful tidbits: Every story closes with useful tidbits for those considering or as of now on their plant-based venture. These pearls of exhortation, brought into the world of individual experience and reflection, are priceless assets for perusers looking for direction and motivation. Whether it's the significance of persistence, the force of local area, or the delight of finding new food varieties and flavors, these bits of knowledge offer consolation and backing to those hoping to roll out enduring improvements.

By sharing these examples of overcoming adversity, this section means to enlighten the fluctuated ways to a plant-based way of life, praising the victories and recognizing the difficulties. These accounts are not simply records of dietary change; they are accounts of self-improvement, further developed wellbeing, and a more profound commitment with the world. They advise us that while the excursion to plant-based living can be testing, it is likewise enormously fulfilling and enhancing, loaded up with revelation, local area, and a restored feeling of direction.

5

Chapter 5: Beyond Nutrition:
The Environmental and Ethical
Impacts

Natural Advantages

The decision of what we put on our plates has sweeping impacts past our own wellbeing, reaching out to the actual soundness of our planet. In this section, we set out on an investigation of the significant ecological advantages that go with the reception of a plant-based diet. The proof is convincing: moving towards an eating regimen wealthy in plants and without any trace of creature items can fundamentally relieve our natural impression, assuming a urgent part in tending to probably the most squeezing ecological issues within recent memory.

Diminishing Carbon Impression: One of the most prompt effects of a plant-based diet is the decrease in ozone harming substance outflows related with food creation. Creature farming is a significant supporter of methane and nitrous oxide emanations, both strong ozone harming substances. By picking plant-based food varieties, which require less energy, land, and water to create, we can definitely cut our carbon impression. This segment dives into the points of interest of how plant-based eats less carbs add to bringing down ozone depleting substance outflows, drawing on logical examination and measurable investigation.

Saving Water: Water shortage is a developing worldwide concern, exacerbated by wasteful and unreasonable farming practices. Animal cultivating is fundamentally more water-escalated than plant cultivating, not just because of the immediate water needs of domesticated animals yet in addition in view of the water expected to develop feed crops. Changing to a plant-based diet can emphatically diminish water utilization, adding to the preservation of this valuable asset. This piece of the section analyzes the water impression of different food varieties, featuring the unmistakable contrasts between plant-based and creature based items.

Safeguarding Area and Biodiversity: The development of rural land for creature touching and feed creation is a main source of deforestation, environment obliteration, and biodiversity misfortune. By taking on a plant-based diet, we lessen the interest for creature items and, thusly, the strain ashore assets. This shift can assist with saving normal territories, safeguard untamed life, and keep up with biodiversity. Through true models and information, this segment outlines the effect of dietary decisions ashore use and biodiversity protection.

In introducing the natural advantages of a plant-based diet, this section means to enlighten the strong association between our food decisions and the strength of our planet. It's a source of inspiration, empowering perusers to think about the more extensive ramifications of their dietary propensities. By picking food varieties that are feeding to our bodies as well as kind to the Earth, we can add to a reasonable future for all occupants of our planet.

Moral Contemplations

As we dive further into the inspirations driving a plant-based way of life, we can't neglect the moral contemplations that constrain numerous to rethink their dietary decisions. This section investigates the ethical components of our food, explicitly zeroing in on the government assistance of animals and the effect of modern animal cultivating rehearses. It welcomes perusers to draw in with the frequently awkward real factors behind the creation of creature based food sources, encouraging a more profound comprehension of the moral ramifications of our dietary decisions.

The Truth of Modern Animal Cultivating: The underpinning of this conversation is a genuine gander at modern creature horticulture — a framework that focuses on productivity and benefit over the government assistance of creatures. Through illustrating practices, for example, industrial facility cultivating, restricted creature taking care of tasks (CAFOs), and the normal utilization of anti-toxins and development chemicals, this part portrays the circumstances under which numerous creatures are raised for food. The objective isn't to stun, however to illuminate, giving a genuine premise to moral contemplations.

The Moral Contention for Plant-Based Eating: Expanding on this comprehension, we investigate the moral contention for embracing a plant-based diet. This isn't tied in with projecting judgment yet about empowering smart reflection on the association between our food decisions and their more extensive ramifications. It's a challenge to think about sympathy and empathy as core values in our dietary choices, perceiving the inborn worth of every single living being and our capacity to pick benevolence and regard over comfort and custom.

The Effect of Our Decisions: Each feast addresses a decision, and this part dives into how selecting plant-based food varieties can be a strong explanation against the mercilessness and double-dealing inborn in a lot of creature horticulture. It's an insistence of the conviction that all animals reserve the privilege to live liberated from misery and abuse. This segment features how individual decisions can add to request driven changes in the food business, possibly prompting better government assistance conditions for creatures.

Exploring Moral Intricacies: At long last, this part recognizes the intricacies and subtleties of moral eating. It resolves inquiries regarding the supportability of elective cultivating strategies, the morals of eating animal items from little, nearby, accommodating ranches, and the potential for mechanical arrangements like lab-developed meat. This segment energizes a decent and nuanced way to deal with moral eating, perceiving that the excursion towards a more merciful eating regimen is private and can take many structures.

By drawing in with the moral contemplations of our dietary decisions, this section expects to give perusers a more profound comprehension of the effect their food can have on their general surroundings. It's an encouragement to adjust our dietary patterns with our qualities, picking ways that mirror our obligation to sympathy, generosity, and moral stewardship of the planet.

Maintainable Eating Practices

In the excursion towards a plant-based way of life, the discussion reaches out past the plate, enveloping how we can support our planet through manageable eating rehearses. This section dives into the more extensive setting of manageability in our food decisions, offering experiences and down to earth guidance for those hoping to limit their natural effect while partaking in a plant-based diet.

Embracing Neighborhood and Occasional Produce: One of the mainstays of supportable eating is picking privately obtained and occasional produce. This approach diminishes the carbon impression related with significant distance food transport and supports neighborhood cultivating networks. It urges perusers to investigate ranchers' business sectors, join local area upheld horticulture (CSA) projects, and even develop their own produce whenever the situation allows. By eating as one with the seasons, we appreciate fresher, more delicious food varieties yet in addition add to a more practical food framework.

Lessening Food Squander: One more basic part of maintainable eating is limiting food squander. This part offers procedures for arranging dinners productively, putting away leafy foods to expand their newness, and imaginatively utilizing extras. It likewise presents the idea of fertilizing the soil natural waste as a way to enhance soil and decrease methane discharges from landfills. By embracing these practices, people can fundamentally diminish their natural impression, transforming waste decrease into a day to day demonstration of ecological stewardship.

Picking Reasonable Bundling: The ecological effect of bundling is a significant thought in economical eating. This part directs perusers in pursuing more eco-accommodating decisions, for example, settling on mass food varieties to decrease bundling waste, choosing items in recyclable or compostable bundling, and bringing reusable sacks, holders, and containers while shopping. These basic movements can significantly affect lessening plastic contamination and preserving assets.

Figuring out the Effect of Food Creation: At long last, this section tends to the significance of grasping the more extensive natural effects of food creation. It examines the job of natural cultivating in decreasing pesticide use, saving biodiversity, and improving soil wellbeing. Moreover, it addresses the water and land effectiveness of plant-based food sources contrasted with creature items, supporting the ecological benefits of a plant-based diet.

By coordinating these maintainable eating rehearses into our regular routines, we can settle on decisions that sustain our bodies as well as our planet. This part enables perusers with the information and devices to pursue informed choices that line up with their ecological qualities, adding to a better, more reasonable world for people in the future.

Local area and Worldwide Effects

As we explore the complexities of embracing a plant-based diet, it's crucial to perceive the far reaching influence our decisions have past private wellbeing and fulfillment. This section investigates the significant local area and worldwide effects of moving towards plant-based eating, enlightening how individual activities add to a bigger story of progress, manageability, and equity.

The Force of Aggregate Decision: The change to plant-based counts calories isn't simply an individual wellbeing choice; it's an aggregate development with the ability to reshape food frameworks on a worldwide scale. This segment features how expanded interest for plant-based items can drive farming practices towards additional maintainable and moral strategies. By picking plant-based choices, we sign to business sectors and policymakers the developing inclination for food frameworks that focus on natural wellbeing and creature government assistance.

Improving Food Security: A huge part of the world's yields is utilized to take care of animals as opposed to individuals, a training that is wasteful as far as calorie transformation and land use. This section examines how a worldwide shift towards plant-based eating could reuse tremendous measures of farming assets to straightforwardly take care of additional individuals, possibly easing food shortage and further developing food security around the world.

Advancing General Wellbeing: The ramifications of broad reception of plant-based eats less carbs stretch out into general wellbeing domains, offering the possibility to decrease the pervasiveness of constant infections related with maximum usage of creature items. This piece of the part inspects how better populaces can prompt diminished medical services costs and a more noteworthy accentuation on preventive consideration, helping society in general.

Rousing People group Commitment and Activism: At long last, this part urges perusers to consider themselves to be influencers inside their networks. It exhibits instances of grassroots activism, local area cultivating, and instructive effort as ways people can advance plant-based living past their own plates. By taking part in local area endeavors, upholding for open plant-based choices in schools, work environments, and public foundations, people can assume a functioning part in molding a more maintainable and evenhanded food scene.

In winding around together the strings of natural stewardship, food equity, and general wellbeing, this part expects to expand the point of view of adopting a plant-based diet. It's a call to perceive the capability of our dietary decisions to add to a bigger story of positive change, moving perusers to embrace the power they hold to influence their general surroundings. Through cognizant eating and dynamic cooperation, we can all in all fashion a way towards a more supportable, just, and sound planet.

6

∽

Chapter 6: Advanced Plant-Based Nutrition

Entire Food sources versus Handled Food sources

In the scene of plant-based sustenance, the qualification between entire food sources and handled food varieties arises as a principal thought for those looking to boost their medical advantages. This part dives into the substance of entire, negligibly handled food sources, pushing for their focal job in an empowering plant-based diet, while likewise tending to the helpful charm and possible disadvantages of handled plant-based other options.

The Ethics of Entire Food sources: At the core of an entire food varieties plant-based diet are organic products, vegetables, entire grains, vegetables, nuts, and seeds in their most regular and raw structure. This segment highlights the nourishing predominance of entire food sources, wealthy in fundamental supplements, fiber, and phytochemicals — intensifies that work synergistically to advance wellbeing and forestall illness. Entire food varieties are the mainstays of ideal sustenance, offering an abundance of advantages including further developed processing, better glucose control, improved heart wellbeing, and a decreased gamble of ongoing infections.

The Proviso of Handled Food sources: While the plant-based food market has extended to incorporate a wide cluster of handled other options, this section reveals insight into the significance of wisdom. Handled plant-based food sources can offer comfort and assortment, yet they frequently accompany added sugars, salt, unfortunate fats, and counterfeit fixings that can diminish the medical advantages of a plant-based diet. The conversation explores through the subtleties of food handling, assisting perusers with understanding how to pursue better decisions that line up with the standards of entire food nourishment.

Systems for Underlining Entire Food varieties: Progressing to an eating regimen fixated on entire food sources requires something other than an information on their advantages — it requests down to earth procedures for integrating these food varieties into day to day existence. This segment gives significant counsel to choosing, planning, and appreciating entire food varieties. From tips on shopping and dinner prep to imaginative thoughts for making entire food varieties the stars of your feasts, this direction means to make entire food, plant-based eating available and agreeable.

Adjusting Comfort and Sustenance: Perceiving the real factors of present day ways of life, this part likewise addresses how to find some kind of harmony between the dietary goals of entire food sources and the accommodation presented by handled food sources. It offers methodologies for settling on informed decisions when handled food sources are important, like perusing names cautiously, picking items with insignificant and unmistakable fixings, and focusing on handled food sources that actually hold a serious level of healthy benefit.

By embracing the standards illustrated in this part, perusers are prepared to explore the range of plant-based food sources with certainty. The accentuation on entire, insignificantly handled food sources not just fills in as the establishment for ideal wellbeing yet additionally cultivates a more profound association with the regular world through the food sources we eat. This part is a demonstration of the force of entire food varieties to support, recuperate, and flourish inside a plant-based way of life.

Superfoods and Practical Food sources

In the domain of plant-based nourishment, superfoods and practical food sources stand apart for their outstanding supplement profiles and potential medical advantages. This section wanders into the captivating universe of these nourishing forces to be reckoned with, offering experiences into how they can brace a plant-based diet, upgrade in general wellbeing, and even forestall specific medical issue.

Characterizing Superfoods and Useful Food sources: At first, we explain what separates superfoods and practical food varieties from the typical passage. While "superfood" is definitely not a logical term, it's generally used to portray food sources especially plentiful in nutrients, minerals, cell reinforcements, and different supplements that can effectively affect our wellbeing. Practical food varieties are those that significantly affect wellbeing past fundamental sustenance; they can advance ideal wellbeing and assist with decreasing the gamble of sickness. Both assume a crucial part in a balanced plant-based diet.

Focus on Plant-Based Superfoods: This part acquaints perusers with an assortment of plant-based superfoods, itemizing their wholesome substance and the medical advantages they offer. From the omega-3 rich flaxseeds and chia seeds to the cancer prevention agent stalwart berries, and the protein-pressed quinoa, we investigate how these food sources add to heart wellbeing, mental capability, and by and large essentialness. Other highlighted superfoods incorporate dim mixed greens, nuts, and vegetables, each praised for their one of a kind commitments to a nutritious eating routine.

Integrating Superfoods into Your Eating routine: Understanding the advantages of superfoods is a certain something; coordinating them into everyday feasts is another. This section gives viable guidance and innovative thoughts for meshing these healthful heroes into your eating routine. Whether it's beginning the day with a berry-stuffed smoothie, improving plates of mixed greens with seeds and nuts, or basing dinners around good grains like quinoa and amaranth, perusers will find how simple and heavenly it tends to be to help their nourishment with superfoods.

The Decent View on Superfoods: While superfoods can offer

concentrated portions of useful supplements, this part accentuates the significance of dietary variety. No single food can give every one of the supplements we want for ideal wellbeing. Consequently, superfoods ought to supplement a changed plant-based diet, not eclipse it. We urge perusers to partake in a large number of entire food sources to guarantee they're getting a wide range of supplements.

Toward the finish of this section, perusers will be furnished with the information to recognize superfoods and utilitarian food sources as well as to capably integrate them into their plant-based eats less. This investigation of superfoods and practical food sources enlightens their capability to improve wellbeing, making them priceless partners chasing after dietary greatness and prosperity.

Dietary Changes for Explicit Medical issue

Exploring the excursion of plant-based nourishment includes not just grasping the fundamentals of a decent eating routine yet additionally perceiving how certain dietary changes can uphold the administration and counteraction of explicit medical issue. This section dives into the remedial capability of a plant-based diet, offering proof based bits of knowledge and viable direction for fitting nourishing admission to address normal wellbeing concerns.

Coronary illness: For people trying to further develop heart wellbeing, this segment frames the significant job of plant-based counts calories in overseeing and forestalling coronary illness. Accentuating food varieties high in fiber, cell reinforcements, and sound fats — like entire grains, nuts, seeds, and salad greens — can essentially decrease risk factors like elevated cholesterol and hypertension. Explicit suggestions incorporate consolidating omega-3 rich flaxseeds and pecans, and limiting admission of added sugars and refined grains.

Diabetes The board: Overseeing glucose levels is pivotal for those with diabetes, and a plant-based diet can be an amazing asset in such manner. This piece of the section features the significance of picking low glycemic record food sources, like vegetables and non-boring vegetables, and makes sense of how the fiber in entire plant food sources can assist with balancing out glucose levels. Recipes and feast arranging tips are given to assist perusers with making adjusted, diabetes-accommodating dinners.

Diminishing Irritation: Constant irritation is at the base of numerous illnesses, yet dietary decisions can assume a huge part in decreasing aggravation. This part centers around mitigating food sources inside a plant-based diet, including turmeric, berries, and dull salad greens, and educates on diminishing admission with respect to handled food varieties and oils that can compound irritation.

Stomach related Wellbeing: For those managing stomach related issues, this part offers direction on enhancing stomach wellbeing through plant-based sustenance. Underscoring fiber-rich food varieties to help a sound stomach microbiome, and integrating matured food sources like sauerkraut and kimchi for their probiotic benefits, can further develop processing and reduce side effects of conditions like IBS.

Every ailment segment is upheld by momentum research and remembers tributes from people who have encountered upgrades for their wellbeing results through dietary changes. Also, normal dietary worries connected with these circumstances, for example, guaranteeing sufficient protein admission for heart wellbeing or overseeing carb consumption for diabetes, are tended to with viable arrangements.

By applying the wholesome changes framed in this part, perusers can figure out how to change their plant-based diet to help generally speaking wellbeing as well as to target and further develop explicit ailments. This customized way to deal with plant-based eating enables people to play a functioning job in their medical services, involving food as medication to mend and flourish.

Competitors on a Plant-Based Diet

The thought that top actual presentation requires creature items is quickly turning into a fantasy of the past. This section is committed to competitors and genuinely dynamic people who decide to fuel their bodies with plant-based sustenance, exposing normal fantasies and giving an exhaustive manual for meeting their extraordinary dietary requirements.

Groundworks of Athletic Sustenance: The part starts by laying out the center parts of a compelling athletic eating regimen — protein for muscle fix and development, starches for energy, fats for perseverance, and different nutrients and minerals for in general wellbeing and recuperation. It stresses the wealth of these supplements in a plant-based diet and diagrams how to consume them in the right extents to help fiery preparation and recuperation.

Protein Methodologies for Plant-Based Competitors: Perceiving protein's vital job in athletic execution, this part dives into plant-based protein sources, like vegetables, tofu, tempeh, quinoa, and nuts. It disperses the fantasy that plant-based proteins are mediocre, introducing systems for consolidating different plant proteins to guarantee a total amino corrosive profile. Pragmatic guidance is given on how much protein to consume in view of the degree of action and the singular's particular objectives.

Sugars and Fats for Energy and Perseverance: Starches are the essential fuel for extreme focus exercises, while fats are fundamental for longer, perseverance based exercises. This piece of the section guides perusers in choosing superior grade, supplement thick sugar sources, similar to entire grains and natural products, and sound fats, like avocados, seeds, and nuts, to advance execution and energy levels all through preparing and contests.

Micronutrients and Hydration: Consideration is likewise given to the basic job of nutrients, minerals, and hydration in athletic execution. Subtleties on key micronutrients, like iron, calcium, vitamin D, and B nutrients, are talked about, alongside their plant-based sources and their significance in supporting energy creation, bone wellbeing, and oxygen transport. Hydration systems previously, during, and after practice are covered to guarantee ideal execution and recuperation.

Reasonable Feast Arranging and Enhancements: The part wraps up with counsel on dinner arranging and timing for competitors, offering test feast designs that take care of different kinds of preparing plans. Furthermore, it addresses when supplementation may be essential, especially for supplements like vitamin B12, vitamin D, and omega-3 unsaturated fats, giving rules to choosing and utilizing supplements securely and actually.

Toward the finish of this part, plant-based competitors and dynamic people will be outfitted with the information and apparatuses to fuel their bodies for ideal execution and recuperation effectively. It fills in as a demonstration of the force of plant-based sustenance in supporting enthusiastic actual work and accomplishing athletic greatness, preparing for another age of competitors who blossom with an eating regimen established in the abundance of the plant realm.

7

Chapter 7: The Future of Food: Trends and Innovations

Plant-Based Patterns

The scene of food is developing quickly, with plant-based eating at the front of this change. This part investigates the powerful patterns that have launch plant-based eats less from specialty to standard, inspecting the powers that have filled their ascent and the ramifications for the fate of food.

The Flood in Ubiquity: lately, plant-based slims down have seen a remarkable flood in notoriety. This shift isn't bound to committed veggie lovers and vegans however reaches out to a wide segment range, including flexitarians who try to diminish their meat utilization without totally killing it. Factors driving this pattern incorporate developing consciousness of the medical advantages related with plant-based eating, ecological worries, and moral contemplations in regards to creature government assistance.

The Development of Plant-Based Choices: As request has developed, so too has the accessibility of plant-based items in eateries, bistros, and stores. Presently not consigned to the edges, plant-put together choices currently highlight unmistakably with respect to menus and racks, offering customers a consistently extending assortment of decisions. From plant-based burgers that intently emulate the taste and surface of meat to a variety of without dairy milks, cheeses, and yogurts, these choices make progressing to plant-based eating more advantageous and pleasant than any other time.

The Impact of Virtual Entertainment and Superstar Supports: Web-based entertainment stages play had a urgent influence in promoting plant-based consumes less calories, filling in as an integral asset for sharing data, recipes, and individual accounts of change. VIP supports have additionally intensified this pattern, with individuals of note across diversion, sports, and even governmental issues upholding for the advantages of plant-based living. These supports have assisted with destroying generalizations and expand the allure of plant-based diets to a more extensive crowd.

Future Expectations: Looking forward, plant-based eating is ready to proceed with its development direction, forming the fate of food in significant ways. Advancements in food science and innovation, alongside expanding customer interest for supportable and morally delivered food, recommend that plant-based diets will assume an undeniably focal part in worldwide food frameworks. This part finishes up with reflections on the capability of plant-based eating to add to a better, more manageable, and caring world, highlighting the meaning of the patterns that have gotten us to this vital second the historical backdrop of food.

Advancements in Plant-Based Cooking

As the plant-based development develops, so too does the scene of plant-based food, advancing with advancements that are changing the culinary world. This section digs into the state of the art improvements in plant-based food sources, highlighting the imagination and innovation driving the making of meat substitutes, sans dairy items, and a plenty of different choices that challenge the customary view of plant-based eating.

The Ascent of Meat Substitutes: Quite possibly of the most remarkable advancement has been the improvement of plant-based meat substitutes that intently copy the taste, surface, and wholesome profile of creature meat. Utilizing fixings like pea protein, soy, and seitan, food researchers have created items that allure for meat-eaters and veggie lovers the same, making the change to plant-based slims down simpler and more agreeable. This part investigates the innovation behind these items, from expulsion strategies that recreate the stringy design of meat to seasoning techniques that accomplish an exquisite, umami-rich taste.

Without dairy Pleasures: The development of sans dairy items reaches out past the customary soy milk and tofu. This part features the venture into a wide cluster of plant-based milks, cheeses, yogurts, and frozen yogurts produced using nuts, oats, peas, and other plant sources. Developments in aging and mixing procedures have brought about items that offer the smooth surface and complex kinds of their dairy partners, taking special care of the lactose prejudiced and sans dairy fans the same.

Entire Food Developments: Past substitutes for creature items, there's a developing accentuation on entire food advancements that commend the intrinsic characteristics of plant fixings. From jackfruit pulled "pork" to mushroom "bacon," this segment grandstands how straightforward fixings can be changed through culinary innovativeness, offering flavorful and nutritious choices that feature the flexibility of plants.

The Eventual fate of Plant-Based Food: As we plan ahead, the opportunities for plant-based cooking appear to be unfathomable. The part closes with a forward-looking viewpoint on how proceeded with development and customer request will shape the up and coming age of plant-based food sources. From progressions in flavor science and supportability to the coordination of worldwide culinary practices, the eventual fate of plant-based cooking is ready to offer different, delectable, and manageable choices for eaters all over the planet.

Through investigating these advancements in plant-based cooking, this section enlightens the dynamic and developing nature of plant-based eating. It praises the innovativeness and inventiveness that are making plant-based eats less more open, charming, and feasible, proclaiming a future where plant-based choices are a standard, essential piece of the culinary scene.

The Job of Innovation in Plant-Based Nourishment

In a time where innovation converges with each part of our lives, its impact on plant-based sustenance is both significant and extraordinary. This part investigates how mechanical advancements are reshaping the manner in which we approach, comprehend, and draw in with plant-based slims down, making it simpler and more compelling for people to embrace and keep up with this way of life.

Wholesome Applications and Advanced Assets: The appearance of cell phone applications and online stages devoted to plant-based nourishment has reformed admittance to data and backing. These computerized devices offer customized feast arranging, nourishing following, and recipes custom-made to individual wellbeing objectives and dietary inclinations. We dig into how these assets enable people to settle on informed dietary decisions, track their admission of fundamental supplements, and find new plant-based food sources and recipes.

Online People group and Informal organizations: Innovation has likewise worked with the development of lively web-based networks where plant-based eaters can find fellowship, trade tips, and offer encounters. From discussions and online entertainment gatherings to web journals and virtual meetups, these computerized spaces offer a feeling of having a place and backing that is significant for those progressing to or supporting a plant-based diet. This segment features the job of these networks in encouraging a worldwide organization of plant-based advocates, working with information trade, and moving aggregate activity towards a more maintainable and moral food framework.

Advancements in Food Innovation: Past friendly and educational innovations, this part looks at the state of the art improvements in food creation that are extending the potential outcomes of plant-based eating. Lab-developed meat, accuracy maturation, and advances in crop development are only a couple of instances of how science and innovation are being tackled to make practical, moral, and nutritious food choices. These advancements vow to address a portion of the natural and moral difficulties related with customary animal horticulture, offering better approaches to create protein-rich food varieties without the requirement for domesticated animals cultivating.

The Eventual fate of Plant-Based Eating: As we look forward, the convergence of innovation and plant-based sustenance holds energizing potential for additional advancements that will make plant-based consumes less calories more available, agreeable, and coordinated into standard food culture. This part theorizes on future innovative advances, from man-made intelligence driven healthful wanting to practical food creation frameworks, that could additionally alter how we source, get ready, and contemplate plant-based food.

From the perspective of innovation, this section illustrates a future where plant-based sustenance is upheld and upgraded by computerized instruments, online networks, and food developments. It highlights the significant job innovation plays in driving the plant-based progress ahead, making it a fundamental piece of our excursion towards better, more practical, and moral dietary patterns.

Building a Local area

The progress to and upkeep of a plant-based way of life is fundamentally enhanced by the presence of a strong local area. This part digs into the pivotal job local area plays in the plant-based development, featuring how aggregate endeavors can enhance mindfulness, availability, and reception of plant-based eats less across assorted populaces and districts.

The Quintessence of Local area: At its center, the idea of local area inside the plant-based development rises above geological limits, making a worldwide organization of people joined by shared values and objectives. This segment investigates the mental and commonsense advantages of having a place with such a local area, from offering profound help and support to sharing information and assets that make plant-based residing more feasible and pleasant.

Shaping Neighborhood and Worldwide Organizations: This part directs perusers through different roads for finding or building plant-based networks, whether locally through cooking classes, potlucks, and local area gardens, or universally by means of online discussions, web-based entertainment gatherings, and virtual occasions. It underlines the significance of comprehensive spaces where everybody from inquisitive newbies to prepared plant-based veterans can track down help, motivation, and brotherhood.

Local area Drives and Activism: Past private help, plant-based networks frequently participate in drives that advance more extensive mindfulness and availability of plant-based slims down. This piece of the section grandstands fruitful local area drove projects, for example, general wellbeing efforts, school nourishment projects, and coordinated efforts with nearby organizations to increment plant-based choices. These models outline how aggregate activity can impact public insight and strategy, establishing conditions where plant-based decisions are standardized and empowered.

The Force of Shared Encounters: Vital to this section is the figuring out that common encounters — whether they include exploring difficulties, commending accomplishments, or basically partaking in plant-based dinners together — produce solid bonds and a feeling of aggregate character. Tributes and stories from different people and networks highlight the groundbreaking effect of these associations, on private excursions as well as on the more extensive objective of cultivating a more reasonable, caring world.

All in all, this part praises the crucial job of local area in the plant-based development. It certifies that while the choice to take on a plant-based diet might be private, the excursion flourishes with shared encounters, common help, and aggregate endeavors. By building and supporting these networks, we can push the plant-based progress ahead, making a gradually expanding influence that advances wellbeing, supportability, and moral living on a worldwide scale.

Conclusion: Embracing the Plant Power Lifestyle

Reflections and Support

As we arrive at the finish of our excursion through "The Plant Power Diet: Change Your Wellbeing with Nature's Abundance," it's critical to stop and ponder the ground we've covered. From the fundamentals of plant-based nourishment to the more extensive ramifications for our well-being, the climate, and society, this book has expected to give a complete manual for taking on a plant-based way of life. Whether you're new to the idea or hoping to extend your responsibility, the excursion towards plant-based living is both individual and significant.

Embracing a plant-based diet is about something other than changing what's on your plate; it's tied in with adding to a better self and a better planet. The proof introduced all through this book highlights the force of plant-based food sources to sustain our bodies, lessen the gamble of persistent infections, and reduction our natural impression. In any case, past the statistical data points lies a straightforward truth: each dinner is a potential chance to pursue decisions that mirror our qualities and yearnings for a superior world.

To the people who are toward the start of this excursion, recall that change doesn't work out by accident more or less. It's a way set apart by picking up, testing, and developing. There will be difficulties, yet in addition triumphs — of all shapes and sizes — that will fuel your inspiration to proceed. To the individuals who have been strolling this way for some time, let this book act as a wake up call of why you began and as motivation to continue to push the limits of what's conceivable with plant-based living.

As you push ahead, convey with you the information that your decisions have power. The choice to embrace plant-based eating is a significant demonstration of taking care of oneself and a declaration of sympathy for our planet and its occupants. Let this be a wellspring of consolation as you explore the highs and lows of changing to and keeping a plant-based diet.

All things being equal, I welcome you to see this not as an end, but rather as the start of a deep rooted experience. The plant-based venture is rich with revelations, flavors, and associations that enhance our lives surprisingly. May you approach each step with interest, transparency, and a feeling of delight in the information that you are essential for a developing development towards a more supportable, stimulating, and sympathetic world.

Proceeding with Your Schooling

As we arrive at the finish of this aide, it's vital to perceive that the excursion toward a plant-controlled way of life doesn't end here. Embracing plant-based living is a persistent course of picking up, developing, and advancing. This part accentuates the significance of promoting your schooling and investigation in the domains of plant-based nourishment, ecological manageability, and moral food decisions.

A Universe of Assets: The plant-based development is upheld by an abundance of information and assets intended to teach and rouse. From thorough sustenance guides and logical examination papers to narratives featuring the ecological and wellbeing effects of our food decisions, there's no deficiency of data to assist with extending your comprehension. This part gives an organized rundown of books, sites, and movies that offer significant bits of knowledge into the advantages and execution of plant-based living.

Long lasting Getting the hang of: Taking on a plant-based way of life is a chance for deep rooted learning. Whether it's remaining refreshed on the most recent dietary exploration, investigating new culinary procedures, or understanding the developing ecological ramifications of food creation, there's continuously a new thing to find. This piece of the part urges perusers to search out courses, studios, and talks — both on the web and face to face — that can improve their insight and abilities.

The Job of Local area in Training: Learning is many times seriously improving and pleasant when imparted to other people. This part features the job of plant-based networks in encouraging training and development. From neighborhood support gatherings and cooking classes to online discussions and web-based entertainment stages, interfacing with similar people can give an abundance of information, encounters, and points of view that improve your plant-based venture.

Strengthening Through Information: At last, proceeding with your schooling in plant-based living is about strengthening. With information comes the capacity to settle on informed decisions that line up with your qualities, add to your wellbeing and prosperity, and effect the world decidedly. This segment closes with a call to embrace the excursion of instruction as a fundamental piece of living a careful, plant-fueled life.

By focusing on continuous instruction and investigation, you outfit yourself with the devices to explore the plant-based way of life unhesitatingly and actually. This part fills in as a scaffold to the following stages in your excursion, empowering you to look for information, challenge presumptions, and fill in manners that enhance your life as well as the existences of people around you and the planet we as a whole offer.

The Source of inspiration

As we end this complete manual for embracing the plant power way of life, it's basic to perceive that the embodiment of this excursion stretches out past the pages of a book. This part is a clarion source of inspiration, encouraging you to lead of plant-based living into your daily existence, as a dietary decision as well as a comprehensive way to deal with wellbeing, supportability, and moral living.

Embracing Plant-Based Living: The initial step is frequently the most huge. Integrating more plant-based food varieties into your eating routine is a significant statement of your obligation to your wellbeing and the prosperity of the planet. This part gives viable tips to slowly expanding your admission of plant-based food sources, proposing straightforward trades, dinner arranging methodologies, and how to explore social circumstances with elegance and certainty.

Backing and Impact: Equipped with information and individual experience, you're in a strong situation to advocate for plant-based living. Whether it's offering your excursion to loved ones, participating in local area conversations, or supporting strategies that advance economical food frameworks, your voice can move change. This piece of the section urges you to track down ways of pushing for plant-based living that resound with your special abilities and interests.

Local area Inclusion: The excursion is more extravagant and more compensating when shared. Engaging in plant-based networks, whether on the web or locally, can offer help, motivation, and amazing open doors for joint effort. This segment investigates different ways of drawing in with and add to these networks, from chipping in at neighborhood food centers to taking part in or coordinating plant-based food occasions.

Having an Effect: Each feast is a potential chance to decide in favor of the sort of world you need to live in. By picking plant-based choices, you add to an interest for more practical, moral, and restorative food decisions. This part closes with a sign of the gradually expanding influence your decisions can have, empowering you to embrace the plant power way of life for yourself, yet for the aggregate fate of our planet.

This source of inspiration is an update that the excursion doesn't end here. It's a continuous course of development, learning, and support. By making these strides, you join a worldwide development of people focused on having an effect, each plant-based decision in turn. Together, we have the ability to change our wellbeing, safeguard our planet, and make a more merciful world.

Affirmations

As we close the pages of this manual for embracing the plant power way of life, it's basic to stop and stretch out our most profound appreciation to the bunch people and networks that have prepared for plant-based living to thrive. This excursion, wealthy in change and revelation, isn't singular. It is a way strolled in the organization of endless supporters, scientists, culinary specialists, and regular people whose commitments have enlightened the way.

Appreciation to the Trailblazers: First, we honor the trailblazers of plant-based sustenance and natural stewardship, whose early exploration and backing laid the foundation for the development we see today. Their commitment to revealing the insights about our food frameworks and their effects on wellbeing and the climate proceeds to motivate and direct us.

Commending the Gourmet experts and Makers: A unique affirmation is because of the imaginative cooks and recipe makers who have changed plant-based fixings into culinary show-stoppers. Their imagination in the kitchen has made plant-based eating nutritious as well as a great experience in taste, testing and changing discernments about what plant-based food can be.

Appreciation for the Scientists and Instructors: Our appreciation reaches out to the specialists and teachers devoted to propelling comprehension we might interpret plant-based sustenance and supportability. Through their thorough work, they give the proof and experiences essential for informed direction, adding to a more educated and engaged local area.

Saying thanks to the Local area: To the dynamic, worldwide local area of plant-based eaters, activists, and promoters — your enthusiasm, support, and shared encounters make an embroidery of motivation that urges others to investigate and embrace this way of life. Your accounts of change and promotion are the heartbeat of this development, driving change each feast in turn.

A Note to the Peruser: In conclusion, however in particular, we recognize you, the peruser. Your interest, receptiveness, and readiness to leave on or proceed with this excursion imply a strong obligation to your wellbeing, the planet, and the prosperity of every one of its occupants. Whether you are toward the start of your plant-based excursion or well along the way, your decisions add to a flood of positive change that stretches out a long ways past your plate.

This book is a demonstration of the aggregate endeavors of a local area joined by a dream of a better, more reasonable, and humane world. As we plan ahead, let us keep on sharing, learn, and develop together, roused by the information that each step we move toward a more brilliant, plant-controlled future.